Human Anatomy: The enigma of love and it's yearnings

by

Marshall Jones

Copyright © 2023 by Marshall Jones

Published by
Jojan press

Library of Congress
Cataloging-in-Publication Data:

Cover design by John Smith

Cover image: © 2023 Marshall Jones

Dedication
To my wife

You have been my unwavering source of love, support, and inspiration throughout this journey. Your encouragement and belief in me have made this book possible. Thank you for being the guiding light in my life.

With all my love,

Marshall Jones.

<u>Table of contents</u>

Introduction

Envision a reality where each pulsating heart is a signal of adoration, and each nerve is a pathway to longing. In this world, the human body isn't simply a complex organic machine, but a guide to the most profound secrets of the human spirit.

This book is an excursion into the human body, investigating the physical and close-to-home underpinnings of affection and want. From the perspective of life structures, we will find how our bodies are wired for association, and how our actual encounters shape our close-to-home ones.

From the shuddering of the heart to the blush of the cheeks, from the flood of adrenaline to the arrival of oxytocin, our bodies are continually conveying our most profound longings. In this book, we will figure out how to pay attention to the language of the body and translate its mysteries.

We will likewise investigate the physical premise of catastrophe, misfortune, and anguish. We will figure out how our bodies answer profound torment, and how we can track down mending amidst it.

At last, this book is a festival of the human body and its uncommon limit with respect to cherish. It is an encouragement to investigate the conundrum of affection and longing

Chapter 1:

A Journey through human anatomy

The study of the composition and arrangement of the human body is known as human anatomy.

The story of human evolution begins with the origins of life on Earth, followed by the emergence of multicellular organisms, leading to the development of complex life forms. For generations, scientists, medical professionals, and inquisitive people have been captivated by the intricate and masterfully designed human body, which is the subject of human anatomy study. This chapter aims to provide a comprehensive understanding of the structure, organization, and interactions among the body's systems by delving deeply into the principles of human anatomy. We will go deeply into the marvel of human anatomy.

The Brain and Emotions: The human brain, with its remarkable complexity and intricacy, is the seat of our emotions, governing the full spectrum of human feelings and behaviors. Emotions, the very essence of our humanity, are deeply intertwined with the brain's structure, function, neurochemistry, and the relationship between the brain and emotions, aiming to unravel the enigmatic nature of our feelings, their neural underpinnings, and their significance in our lives.

The limbic system:

The limbic system is a complex set of brain structures that play a crucial role in regulating emotions, memory, and various aspects of behavior. It is sometimes referred to as the "emotional brain" or "emotional center" of the brain because of its significant involvement in emotional processing and the formation of emotional memories. The limbic system is not a single isolated structure but rather a network of interconnected regions within the brain.

Key components of the limbic system include

the hippocampus: The hippocampus is involved in the formation and consolidation of long-term memories, particularly declarative and episodic memories. It plays a vital role in spatial navigation and cognitive mapping.

Amygdala: The amygdala is primarily associated with processing emotions, especially fear and threat detection. It plays a critical role in evaluating the emotional significance of stimuli and in the formation of emotional memories.

Cingulate Cortex: The cingulate cortex is involved in various cognitive functions, including emotional regulation, pain perception, and decision-making. It helps mediate emotional responses and assess the emotional salience of stimuli.

Mammillary Bodies: The mammillary bodies are involved in memory, particularly emotional memory. They are connected to the hippocampus and other brain structures, contributing to the formation of emotional memories.

Hypothalamus: The hypothalamus is crucial for maintaining physiological balance, regulating various bodily functions, and responding to emotional cues. It controls the autonomic nervous system, influencing stress responses, temperature regulation, and feeding behaviors.

The limbic system's interconnected nature allows it to play a central role in processing emotions, forming emotional memories, and influencing various aspects of behavior and cognition. It is not isolated from the rest of the brain but rather interacts with other brain regions to regulate emotional responses and adaptive behaviors.

The limbic system is a key player in mood disorders, anxiety disorders, addiction, and post-traumatic stress disorder (PTSD) when it functions abnormally. Understanding the limbic system is crucial for grasping the neurological underpinnings of emotions, memory, and various clinical conditions related to emotional and cognitive dysregulation.

The brain stem:

The brainstem is a critical region of the brain that plays a fundamental role in regulating many of our basic physiological functions and is indirectly involved in emotional processing. To understand the connection between the brainstem and emotions, it's essential to explore the brainstem's structure and its influence on various aspects of emotional experiences. The brainstem is located at the base of the brain and connects the brain to the spinal cord. It consists of three main parts:

Medulla Oblongata: The lowest part of the brainstem, the medulla oblongata, controls essential autonomic functions like heart rate, breathing, blood pressure, and digestion. While it's not directly involved in emotional processing, disruptions in these vital functions can affect emotional well-being.

Pons: Located just above the medulla, the pons serve as a bridge connecting different regions of the brain. It's involved in sleep and arousal, respiration, and the relay of sensory information. While the pons contribute to emotional stability through their role in regulating arousal and alertness, it's not primarily responsible for emotional processing.

Midbrain (Mesencephalon): The midbrain, situated above the pons, plays a more indirect but significant role in emotional responses. It contains the reticular formation, a complex network of neurons that regulates consciousness, alertness, and the sleep-wake cycle. This part of the brainstem helps control emotional reactions by influencing one's overall state of arousal and vigilance

Neurotransmitters:

Various neurotransmitters, such as serotonin, dopamine, and

norepinephrine, play a significant role in mood regulation and emotional stability. Imbalances in these neurotransmitters can lead to mood disorders like depression and anxiety

Hormones:

Hormones, like cortisol and oxytocin, are released in response to emotional situations and can affect emotional states. For example, cortisol is linked to the stress response, while oxytocin is associated with bonding and social attachment

Cortisol: Cortisol is often referred to as the "stress hormone." It is released in response to stressful situations and helps the body prepare for a fight-or-flight response. While cortisol is essential for survival, chronically high levels of cortisol can lead to anxiety, depression, and other mood disorders.

Oxytocin: Often called the "love hormone" or "bonding hormone," oxytocin is associated with social bonding, trust, and emotional connections. It is released during activities such as hugging, cuddling, and intimate moments, promoting feelings of attachment and closeness.

Serotonin: Serotonin is a neurotransmitter that also acts as a hormone. It plays a critical role in regulating mood and emotions. Low serotonin levels are linked to conditions like depression and anxiety. Medications known as selective serotonin reuptake inhibitors (SSRIs) are commonly used to increase serotonin levels and alleviate symptoms of these disorders.

Dopamine: While dopamine is primarily a neurotransmitter, it is involved in feelings of pleasure and reward. It is often associated with positive emotions, motivation, and reinforcement. Dysregulation of dopamine can contribute to mood disorders like depression and addiction.

Norepinephrine: Norepinephrine, another neurotransmitter that also acts as a hormone, is associated with the body's fight-or-flight response. It helps in increasing alertness and focus during stressful or dangerous situations. Abnormal levels of norepinephrine can contribute to conditions like anxiety and post-traumatic stress disorder (PTSD).

Endorphins: Endorphins are often called "feel-good" hormones. They are released during activities like exercise, laughter, and even pain. Endorphins act as natural painkillers and can produce a sense of euphoria and well-being.

Progesterone and Estrogen: These sex hormones, primarily found in higher levels in women, can influence mood and emotional states. Changes in oestrogen and progesterone levels during the menstrual cycle can lead to premenstrual syndrome (PMS) and mood fluctuations.

Testosterone: While predominantly a male hormone, testosterone is also present in smaller quantities in females. It can influence aggression and assertiveness, which can affect emotional responses.

Sexual dimorphism: Sexual dimorphism refers to the differences in physical characteristics, such as size, shape, and colour, between males and females of a species. These differences are typically related to the distinct roles and functions that males and females have in reproduction and other aspects of their biology. These differences in physical traits often arise due to the specific evolutionary pressures and roles that each sex has in reproduction and survival. For example, in species where males compete for access to females, males may evolve traits that help them win these competitions, such as larger body size or weaponry. Females, on the other hand, may evolve traits that enhance their ability to care for and protect offspring. Sexual dimorphism is a fascinating aspect of biology and can vary significantly from one species to another. It is a result of natural selection and sexual selection, where certain traits are favored because they increase an individual's chances of successfully reproducing and passing on their genes to the next generation.

The heart and love: The concept of love, often associated with strong emotional and psychological experiences, has a fascinating connection to the human heart and its anatomy. While love is primarily a complex emotion, the heart plays a significant symbolic and physiological role in this context.

Physiological Responses: Love and emotions can trigger physiological responses that involve the heart. For instance, when people experience intense emotions such as love or attraction, their heart rate may increase. This is due to the release of adrenaline and other stress hormones, which prepare the body for action. These responses can be related to the fight-or-flight reaction, which is connected to the heart's functioning.

Oxytocin and Bonding: The hormone oxytocin, often called the "love hormone" or "bonding hormone," plays a role in emotional connections and social bonding. Oxytocin release can be stimulated through physical touch, like hugging or kissing, and it contributes to feelings of closeness and attachment.

Brain-Heart Connection: Love is primarily a product of brain activity and complex neural processes. The brain processes emotions, including love, and sends signals to the heart to regulate its activity. This connection between the brain and the heart is a central aspect of the emotional experience.

Physical Sensations: Strong emotions, such as love and excitement, can lead to physical sensations in the chest, often described as "feeling one's heart race" or "having one's heart skip a beat." These sensations are due to changes in heart rate driven by the release of hormones like adrenaline during emotional experiences.

In summary, the heart's symbolic association with love stems from the physical sensations people feel during emotionally charged moments. While the heart's anatomy is essential for circulatory function, the emotion of love is a complex interplay of various factors, primarily rooted in the brain and emotional experiences, rather than the physical anatomy of the heart.

Chapter2:

Beyond the Bones

The anatomy of the human body can play a role in the experience of romance and love, particularly in how it influences a person's physical responses and sensations during these emotional states. In light of romance and love, consider the following considerations about how a person's anatomy affects them.

Neurobiology of Love: Certain brain mechanisms are linked to feelings of love and romantic attraction. Feelings of attachment and pleasure linked with love are partly attributed to the release of hormones such as dopamine and oxytocin in the brain.

Bodily Sensations: A person experiencing love or infatuation may experience a range of bodily feelings, such as an elevated heart rate, butterflies in the stomach, and an adrenaline rush. These feelings are connected to the body's "fight or flight" reaction and are caused by modifications in the autonomic nerve system.

Facial Expressions: The anatomy of facial muscles plays a role in the non-verbal communication of love and affection. Smiles, eye contact, and facial expressions are often used to convey romantic interest and affection.

Sense of Touch: The body's sense of touch and the anatomy of the skin are crucial in romantic relationships. Physical touch, such as hugging, kissing, and holding hands, can elicit feelings of warmth and closeness

Sensory Perception: The senses of sight, smell, and hearing are involved in the perception of romantic partners. Physical appearance, scent, and the sound of a loved one's voice can all contribute to feelings of attraction and love.

Health Effects: Love and positive romantic relationships have been associated with various health benefits, including reduced stress, improved heart health, and enhanced overall well-being. These effects are attributed to the release of certain hormones and the reduction of stress hormones in the body.

Sexual Anatomy: In romantic and intimate relationships, the anatomy of sexual organs is significant. The physical aspects of sexual attraction and intimacy are closely tied to the anatomy of genitalia and reproductive systems.

Anatomical variations and their impact on human sexuality

Anatomical variations in human sexuality are relatively common and can affect both men and women. Some of the most common variations include

Variations in the clitoris: The clitoris is the primary organ of female sexual pleasure, and it can vary in size, shape, and location. Some women have clitorises that are buried under the skin, while others have clitorises that are more prominent. The clitoris can also be located closer to the front or back of the vagina.

Variations in the vagina: The vagina is a muscular tube that connects the uterus to the outside of the body. It can vary in length, width, and depth. Some women have vaginas that are shorter or narrower than others. The vagina can also be more or less curved.

Variations in the uterus: The uterus is a pear-shaped organ that is located in the lower abdomen. It houses the developing fetus during pregnancy. The uterus can vary in size, shape, and position. Some women have uteruses that are tilted forward or backward. The uterus can also be more or less flexible.

Variations in the penis: The penis is the male organ of reproduction. It can vary in size, shape, and curvature. Some men have penises that are shorter or thinner than others. The penis can also be more or less curved.

Variations in the testes: The testes are the male reproductive organs. They are located in the scrotum, which is a sac of skin that hangs below the penis. The testes can vary in size, shape, and position. Some men have testes that are smaller or larger than others. The testes can also be more or less descended, meaning that they may be closer to the body or hang lower.

Variations in the labia: The labia are the folds of skin that surround the vagina and clitoris. They can vary in size, shape, and thickness. Some women have labia that are larger or smaller than others. The labia can also be more or less wrinkled.

These are just a few of the many anatomical variations that can affect human sexuality. Most of these variations are harmless and do not affect a person's ability to have sex or experience pleasure. However, some variations can cause problems, such as pain during sex or difficulty getting pregnant. If you are concerned about an anatomical variation, it is important to talk to a doctor or other healthcare provider.

It is important to remember that everyone is different, and there is no one "normal" body. Anatomical variations are a part of human diversity and should be celebrated.

Anatomical challenges and intimacy;

Physical difficulties can influence closeness in different ways, influencing both physical and profound parts of a relationship. These difficulties can emerge from a scope of elements, including actual handicaps, constant sicknesses, surgeries, or normal changes in the body because of maturing or pregnancy.

Actual Intimacy Physical difficulties can straightforwardly influence actual closeness, influencing sexual capabilities, solace during actual friendship, and the capacity to partake in specific exercises. For example, people with spinal line wounds might encounter muscle spasticity or loss of sensation, which can make sex or other actual touch awkward or troublesome. Moreover, certain medical procedures or ailments can prompt changes in the body's life structures, like the passing of an appendage or the presence of scars or embeds. These progressions can influence an individual's mental self-view and certainty, making them reluctant to participate in actual closeness.

Profound Intimacy Physical difficulties can likewise in a roundabout way influence closeness by influencing an individual's personal prosperity and confidence. The anxiety toward dismissal, the sensation of being unique, or the kind of overseeing physical or profound impediments can prompt tension, misery, or a feeling of disconnection. These close-to-home worries can frustrate open correspondence, trust, and weakness, which are pivotal parts of profound closeness.

Tending to Physical Difficulties in Intimacy Exploring physical difficulties in closeness requires open correspondence, understanding, and adaptability from the two accomplices. Open correspondence permits couples to examine their interests, fears, and inclinations transparently, encouraging a feeling of help and acknowledgment.

Understanding and sympathy are fundamental to seeing the value in one another's points of view and constraints, advancing compassion and common regard. Adaptability permits couples to adjust their personal practices to oblige their actual necessities and inclinations, guaranteeing common delight and fulfillment.

Looking for Support In the event that physical difficulties are altogether affecting closeness and connections, looking for proficient help can be gainful.

Specialists or sex advisors can give aaaaaadirection and strategies to improve correspondence, address profound worries, and investigate elective ways of communicating closeness. Moreover, support gatherings can offer a place of refuge for people and couples to share their encounters, get approval, and gain from other people who have confronted comparable difficulties.

Keep in mind, that closeness isn't exclusively about actual touch or sexual action. It envelops profound association, shared encounters, and common regard.

By getting it and tending to physical difficulties, couples can track down ways of keeping up with and developing their closeness in a manner that is significant and satisfying for the two of them.

Immune responses and attraction:

The resistant framework assumes a part in human fascination by impacting the view of fragrance, mate choice, and contraceptive achievement. Studies have shown that people will quite often be more drawn to individuals who have an alternate invulnerable framework from their own. This is on the grounds that the variety in resistant qualities can prompt the development of various significant histocompatibility complex (MHC) particles, which are proteins that assume a part in safe acknowledgment. Individuals with various MHC profiles are bound to have posterity with hereditarily different safe frameworks, which might be gainful for the endurance of the posterity despite assorted microbes.

Aroma and Attraction: The insusceptible framework additionally impacts human fascination through aroma. The body delivers an assortment of odorants, including some that are impacted by MHC particles. Studies have shown that individuals are more drawn to the aroma of individuals with various MHC profiles of their own. This recommends that the resistant framework might assume a part in flagging similarity and conceptive potential.

Mate Choice and Contraceptive Success As well as impacting fragrance and fascination: the resistant framework may likewise assume a part in mate determination and conceptual achievement. Studies have shown that individuals are bound to pick mates who have different MHC profiles from their own. This proposes that the resistant framework might be engaged with mate determination choices and that individuals might be unknowingly picking mates who are probably going to create posterity with solid invulnerable frameworks.

Physical Considerations: no The safe framework likewise assumes a part in human life structures. For instance, the resistant framework is associated with the improvement of the auxiliary sexual qualities that are related with appeal, for example, facial evenness and body shape. Moreover, the safe framework is associated with the creation of chemicals that impact the sexual way of behaving and want.

In general, the resistant framework assumes a complicated and significant part in human fascination. By impacting fragrance, mate determination, and regenerative achievement, the insusceptible framework assists with guaranteeing that people are drawn to mates who are probably going to create solid offspring.

It is essential to take note that the connection between the invulnerable framework and human fascination is complicated and not completely perceived. Further exploration is expected to completely comprehend the components by which the safe framework impacts fascination and mate choice.

Anatomy and aging (sexual health later in life):

Life structures and maturing can influence sexuality in various ways.

Physical changes:

As we age, our bodies go through various actual changes that can influence our sexuality. These progressions can include

Changes in chemical levels: Chemicals assume a critical part in sexual capability. As we age, our chemical levels can decline, which can prompt changes in drive, excitement, and climax.

Changes in the contraceptive organs: The regenerative organs can likewise change with age. For instance, the vagina might become drier and less versatile, and the uterus might recoil. These progressions can make sex less agreeable or even agonising.

Changes in general health: By and large well-being can likewise assume a part in sexual capability. Conditions like diabetes, coronary illness, and joint pain can all influence sexual capability.

Mental changes:

Notwithstanding actual changes, we may likewise encounter mental changes as we age. These progressions can include

Changes in self-image: As we age, we might turn out to be more hesitant about our bodies. This can make it hard to feel great and sure during sex.

Changes in pressure levels: Stress can likewise influence sexual capability. Assuming we are feeling anxious, we might be less intrigued by sex or experience issues becoming excited.

Changes in relationships: Our connections can likewise change as we age. For instance, we might turn out to be more far off from our accomplices or possess less energy for closeness.

In spite of these changes, it is vital to recall that sex can be a pleasurable and satisfying aspect of life at any age.

Here are a few ways to keep a sound sexual coexistence as you age:

- *Speak with your accomplice about your requirements and wants.*

- *Be patient and understanding with one another.*

- *Investigate better approaches to be close.*

- *Look for clinical exhortation on the off chance that you are encountering any issues with your sexual well-being.*

It is likewise vital to recollect that everybody encounters maturing in an unexpected way. Certain individuals might find that their sexual coexistence ages gracefully, while others might find that it declines. There is no set-in-stone manner to encounter sex as you age.

Sexual orientation and identity:

Sexual orientation and identity are complex and multifaceted concepts that encompass a range of feelings and experiences related to one's sexuality and gender. They are often used interchangeably, but there are important distinctions between the two.

Sexual orientation refers to the romantic and/or sexual attraction that a person feels towards others. It is typically categorised as heterosexual (attraction to people of a different sex), homosexual (attraction to people of the same sex), bisexual (attraction to people of both sexes), and asexual (no sexual attraction to anyone).

Sexual identity is a person's internal sense of being male, female, neither, both, or somewhere else on the gender spectrum. It is often expressed through a person's gender expression, which refers to how they present themselves to the world in terms of their clothing, hairstyle, mannerisms, and other outward behaviors.

Gender identity and sexual orientation are not always the same. A person can be a transgender man (born female but identifies as male) who is attracted to women (heterosexual), or a cisgender woman (born female and identifies as female) who is attracted to women (lesbian).

Sexual orientation and sexual identity are also not static; they can evolve over time as a person experiences life and develops their understanding of themselves. Some people may identify as one thing at one point in their lives and then identify as something else later on.

Gender identity and sexual orientation are important aspects of a person's identity, and they can have a significant impact on their lives. It is important to be respectful of the identities of others, even if they are different from our own.

Chapter3:

From Cells to Emotions

The connection between cells and feelings is a perplexing and interesting one that is as yet being investigated by researchers. While there is no immediate coordinated correspondence between cells and feelings, there is developing proof that cell processes assume a part in the age of feelings.

One manner by which cells can add to feelings is through the arrival of synapses. Synapses are synthetic compounds that communicate signals between neurons, or nerve cells. A few synapses, like dopamine, serotonin, and norepinephrine, are known to assume a part in controlling state of mind and conduct. For instance, dopamine is related to joy and reward, while serotonin is related to temperament and prosperity. Norepinephrine is associated with the instinctive reaction and can add to sensations of nervousness and dread.

One more manner by which cells can add to feelings is through the guideline of quality articulation. Quality articulation is the interaction by which qualities are converted into proteins, which are the structure blocks of cells. Various qualities are communicated in various cells, and the example of quality articulation can be changed in light of natural improvements, like pressure or chemicals. This can prompt changes in the way of behaving of cells, which can thus affect feelings.

For instance, one investigation discovered that pressure can prompt changes in the statement of qualities that direct the safe framework. These progressions can make the body more powerless against disease, which can thus prompt sensations of weariness, peevishness, and discouragement.

Notwithstanding the immediate impacts of cell processes on feelings, cells can likewise by implication influence feelings by affecting different frameworks in the body, like the endocrine framework and the autonomic sensory system. The endocrine framework is liable for the creation of chemicals, which are synthetic compounds that move through the circulation system and can influence a large number of physical processes, including feelings. The autonomic sensory system is liable for controlling programmed physical processes, for example, pulse and circulatory strain. Stress can initiate the autonomic sensory system, which can prompt sensations of tension and dread.

By and large, obviously cells assume a mind-boggling and significant part in the age of feelings. While there is still a lot to find out about this relationship, researchers are proceeding to gain ground in understanding how cells add to our profound encounters. The many-sided dance of cells assumes a significant part in molding our ability for affection, impacting the actual articulations of love as well as the more profound close-to-home embroidery of our connections. Understanding the cell systems' hidden love gives an interesting look into the organic underpinnings of this mind-boggling human inclination.

Neurotransmitters: The Substance Couriers of Love

Love's ensemble is coordinated by a fountain of synapses, the substance couriers that hand off data between neurons in the mind. These particles, working in the show, shape our profound scene, impacting our sensations of connection, closeness, and holding.

Among the central members in this brain symphony is oxytocin, frequently named the "affection chemical." Emitted by the nerve center, a district profound inside the cerebrum, oxytocin advances sensations of trust, sympathy, and social holding. It assumes a significant part in mother-baby holding, match holding, and, surprisingly, social acknowledgment.

Vasopressin, another neuropeptide, accomplishes with oxytocin to fortify the powers of profound devotion. It upgrades pair-holding, advances specific hostility with regard to friends and family, and adds to the arrangement of long-haul recollections related to adoration and connection.

Dopamine, the synapse related to delight and reward, likewise adds to the affection experience. It fills the happiness and fervor frequently connected with heartfelt love, building up the pleasurable parts of connections.

Serotonin, another synapse, assumes a more unobtrusive yet critical part enamored. It manages mindset, impulsivity, and hostility, adding to the steadiness and security that support enduring connections.

Hormones: The Body's Affection Language

Past the domain of synapses, chemicals, and the body's substance communicators, likewise impact our ability for affection. Testosterone, the essential male sex chemical, advances predominance, animosity, and cutthroat way of behaving. Nonetheless, it likewise adds to coordinate holding and the craving for closeness.

Oestrogen, the essential female sex chemical, advances sustaining, compassion, and social holding. It assumes a part in managing the monthly cycle and can impact sexual craving and responsiveness.

The Job of Mind Areas in Love;
The unpredictable embroidery of adoration is woven by an organization of cerebrum locales, each contributing remarkable strings to the general insight. The ventral tegmental region

(VTA), found profound inside the midbrain, fills in as a prized community, delivering dopamine and building up sure encounters, incorporating those related to adoration and love.

The core accumbens, one more central member in the award framework, gets dopamine from the VTA and coordinates signals from different mind locales, incorporating those engaged with feeling and inspiration. It assumes a part in the expectation and experience of joy, adding to the habit-forming nature of heartfelt love.

The prefrontal cortex, the mind's chief control community, directs feelings, channels interruptions, and decides. It is engaged with assessing likely accomplices, surveying similarity, and settling on decisions that advance long-haul connections.

The Effect of Life Encounters on Love

While our science gives the establishment to our ability for adoration, it is our background that shapes and refine this capacity. Youth encounters, especially those including connection and security, lay the preparation for future connections. Positive early associations cultivate trust, sympathy, and the capacity to shape secure bonds, while pessimistic encounters can prompt close-to-home separation and trouble with closeness.

Over the course of life, our encounters with adoration and misfortune keep on forming our profound scene. Positive encounters support our ability for adoration, while disaster and selling out can prompt apprehension about weakness and trouble confiding in others.

Conclusion

Love, in the entirety of its intricacy and magnificence, is a result of complex natural cycles that unfurl inside our cells and cerebrum districts. Synapses, chemicals, and brain networks arrange the ensemble of feelings, while our background shapes and refines our capacity to frame and support cherishing connections.

Understanding the organic underpinnings of adoration gives a captivating look into the profundities of human inclination, uncovering the fragile dance between our science and our encounters in molding our ability for adoration.

Chapter4:

Love's biological blueprint

Love, the most significant and complex of human feelings, has for quite some time been a subject of interest and discussion. Writers, savants, and researchers the same have tried to figure out its temperament and starting points, yet it remains a riddle.

As of late, in any case, researchers have started to unwind the natural underpinnings of adoration, uncovering a perplexing exchange of chemicals, synapses, and cerebrum structures that underlie our ability for profound association and love.

Hormones: The Compound Couriers of Affection

Chemicals, the body's compound communicators, assume a basic part in molding our profound scene, including our encounters of adoration. Oxytocin, frequently named the "affection chemical," is a neuropeptide created by the nerve center and emitted into the circulatory system. It is related to sensations of trust, compassion, and social holding, and assumes a critical part in mother-newborn child holding, match holding, and, surprisingly, social acknowledgment.

Vasopressin, another neuropeptide, accomplishes with oxytocin to fortify the powers of profound devotion. It upgrades pair-holding, advances specific animosity with regard to friends and family, and adds to the arrangement of long-haul recollections related to adoration and connection.

Dopamine, a synapse related to delight and prize, likewise adds to the adoration experience. It energizes the rapture and energy frequently connected with heartfelt love, building up the pleasurable parts of connections.

Serotonin, another synapse, assumes a more unobtrusive yet critical part infatuated. It directs mindset, impulsivity, and animosity, adding to the dependability and security that support enduring connections.

Cerebrum Locales: The Brain Hardware of Adoration

The perplexing embroidery of affection is woven by an organization of mind districts, each contributing extraordinary strings to the general insight. The ventral tegmental region (VTA), found profound inside the midbrain, fills in as a prized community, delivering dopamine and supporting positive encounters, incorporating those related to affection and friendship.

The prefrontal cortex, the cerebrum's chief control community, directs feelings, channels interruptions, and decides. It is engaged with assessing possible accomplices, surveying similarity, and settling on decisions that advance long-haul connections.

Valuable Encounters: Moulding Our Ability for Affection

While our science gives the establishment to our ability for affection, it is our background that shapes and refines this capacity. Youth encounters, especially those including connection and security, lay the basis for future connections. Positive early connections cultivate trust, compassion, and the capacity to shape secure bonds, while pessimistic encounters can prompt profound separation and trouble with closeness.

Over the course of life, our encounters with affection and misfortune keep on forming our close-to-home scene. Positive encounters support our ability for adoration, while catastrophe and selling out can prompt feelings of dread toward weakness and trouble confiding in others.

Conclusion: Love's Organic Outline

Love, in the entirety of its intricacy and magnificence, is a result of mind-boggling natural cycles that unfurl inside our cells and cerebrum locales. Synapses, chemicals, and brain networks organize the ensemble of feelings, while our background shape and refine our capacity to frame and support adoring connections.

Understanding the organic underpinnings of adoration gives a captivating look into the profundities of human inclination, uncovering the sensitive dance between our science and our encounters in molding our ability for adoration.

The cingulate cortex: The cingulate cortex is a huge, complex cerebrum locale that assumes a part in a large number of capabilities, including

Feeling guidelines: The cingulate cortex is engaged with directing our feelings, including love. It assists us with controlling our feelings and communicating them in a sound manner.

Torment insight: The cingulate cortex is additionally associated with torment discernment. It assists us with interpreting and answering torment signals.

Decision-making: The cingulate cortex is associated with navigation. It assists us with gauging the upsides and downsides of various choices and pursuing decisions that are to our greatest advantage.

Motivation: The cingulate cortex is associated with inspiration. It assists us with keeping fixed on our objectives and conquering obstructions.

The cingulate cortex is separated into two primary parts: the foremost cingulate cortex (ACC) and the back cingulate cortex (PCC). The ACC is engaged with additional prompt feelings, like love, while the PCC is associated with additional intricate feelings, like compassion.

How the Cingulate Cortex Connects with Affection

The cingulate cortex is remembered to assume a part enamoured in more ways than one. In the first place, it is associated with the experience of remuneration and delight. At the point when we are enamoured, our minds discharge dopamine, a synapse that is related to remuneration and joy. This dopamine discharge is remembered to add to the euphoric and invigorating sentiments that are frequently connected with heartfelt love.

Second, the cingulate cortex is engaged with consideration and concentration. At the point when we are infatuated, our cerebrums become more centered around the individual we love. This is believed to be expected to some degree to expand action in the cingulate cortex.

Third, the cingulate cortex is associated with sympathy. At the point when we are enamored, we are better ready to comprehend and talk about the thoughts of the individual we love. This is believed to be expected to some extent to expand movement in the cingulate cortex.

Concentrates on the Cingulate Cortex and Love

Various examinations have shown that the cingulate cortex is actuated when individuals are enamored. For instance, one investigation discovered that the cingulate cortex was more dynamic in individuals who were shown photos of their friends and family than in individuals who were shown pictures of outsiders.

Another investigation discovered that the cingulate cortex was more dynamic in individuals who were in another heartfelt connection than in individuals who were in a drawn-out relationship. This proposes that the cingulate cortex might be more dynamic in the beginning phases of affection when we are encountering the most extreme sensations of fascination and enthusiasm.

In conclusion,

The cingulate cortex is a mind boggling and significant cerebrum district that assumes a part enamoured. It is engaged with managing our feelings, concentrating, and understanding and talking about the thoughts of the individual we love.

Chapter5:

Chemistry Comes Alive

Experiencing passionate feelings is a complicated and complex peculiarity that has enamored the minds of writers, savants, and researchers for a really long time. While there is no single meaning of affection or a generally settled upon clarification for why it happens, specialists have gained huge headway in understanding the natural, mental, and social factors that add to this significant human experience.

Organic Underpinnings of Love:

The experience of affection is well established in our science, with different chemicals and synapses assuming a significant part in the close-to-home and actual sensations related to it. Oxytocin, frequently named the "affection chemical," is a neuropeptide that advances sensations of trust, compassion, and social holding. It is delivered during actual touch, like embracing or kissing, and is remembered to add to the feeling of connection and closeness that describes heartfelt love.

Dopamine, one more synapse related to delight and prize, is likewise associated with the affection experience. It builds up good ways of behaving, incorporating those related with adoration and friendship, and adds to the happiness and energy frequently felt in the beginning phases of close connections.

Serotonin, a synapse that controls the state of mind and impulsivity, assumes a more unobtrusive yet critical part enamored. It adds to the soundness and security that support enduring connections.

Mental Parts of Love:

Mentally, love includes a scope of feelings, considerations, and ways of behaving. Energetic love is described by extreme sensations of fascination, fervor, and yearning for the dearest. Conversely, companionate love is portrayed by sensations of closeness, security, and connection.

Love likewise includes mental cycles, like admiration, by which we trait positive characteristics to our accomplices, and attribution inclination, by which we decipher their activities all the better. These cycles can add to the support of adoration by building up our positive impression of our accomplices.

Social and Social Effects on Love:

Love isn't exclusively a result of science and brain research; it is likewise moulded by friendly and social elements. Our encounters with family, companions, and society impact how we might interpret love and how we express it. Social standards and assumptions can likewise play a part in the development and articulation of affection connections.

Phases of Love:

While affection is a dynamic and consistently developing experience, it tends to be comprehensively partitioned into three phases:

Infatuation: Described by extreme sensations of energy, fervour, and glorification.

Attraction: Portrayed by developing sensations of closeness, trust, and connection.

Commitment: Described by a profound and persevering through bond, frequently joined by long-haul plans for the relationship.

Challenges and Keeping up with Love:

In spite of its many advantages, love can likewise introduce difficulties. Captivation can blur, fascination can melt away, and struggle can emerge. Keeping up with adoration requires exertion, correspondence, and an eagerness to adjust and become together.

Love as an All-inclusive Human Experience

In spite of the variety of human societies and encounters, love is a widespread human feeling that has been perceived across societies since the beginning of time. A strong power interfaces us with other people, gives us a feeling of having a place and security, and can propel us to act with graciousness, empathy, and liberality.

Understanding the natural, mental, and social underpinnings of affection can assist us with better valuing its intricacies and exploring the difficulties that emerge in connections. It can likewise give a more profound appreciation of the significant effect that affection has on our day-to-day routines and the existence of everyone around us.

Sexual responses and anatomy*:* Sexual reaction is a complex physiological cycle that includes various changes in the body. These progressions are ordinarily separated into four phases:

Fervour **:** The fervor stage is described by an expansion in the bloodstream to the privates, expansion of the privates, and grease of the vagina (in ladies). In men, the penis becomes erect. The energy stage is regularly brought about by sexual excitement, which can be set off by various improvements, like actual touch, dream, or viewable signals.

Level: The level stage is portrayed by a continuation of the progressions that started in the energy stage. In ladies, the grease of the vagina proceeds, and the clitoris turns out to be more delicate. In men, the erection of the penis proceeds, and the balls become engorged with blood. The level stage is normally the longest phase of the sexual reaction cycle.

Climax: Climax is the pinnacle of sexual delight. It is portrayed by a progression of compulsory muscle compressions in the private parts and pelvis. In ladies, the climax is regularly joined by a compression of the clitoris and vaginal muscles. In men, climax is regularly joined by discharge, the removal of semen from the penis.

Resolution: The resolution stage is characterized by a gradual return to the body's pre-arousal state. The genitals return to their normal size and blood flow decreases. The resolution stage can last for several minutes or longer.

Life systems of the sexual organs

The sexual organs are the organs that are associated with sexual propagation and sexual joy. The sex organs are different for people.

Male sexual organs

The male sexual organs include

Penis: The penis is the male sex organ utilised for sex and pee. Composed of spongy tissue that loads up with blood during an erection.

Testicles: The balls are the male regenerative organs. They produce sperm and testosterone, the male sex chemical.

Scrotum: The scrotum is a sac of skin that holds the balls.

Urethra: The urethra is a cylinder that stores urine and semen of the body.

The female sexual organs include:

Vagina: The vagina is a solid cylinder that leads from an external perspective of the body to the cervix. It is utilised for sex, labour, and period.

Clitoris: The clitoris is a little, touchy organ that is situated at the front of the vagina. It is the essential wellspring of sexual joy in ladies.

Labia majora: The labia majora are two folds of skin that encompass the vagina and clitoris. They are canvassed in pubic hair.

Labia minora: The labia minora are two more modest folds of skin that are situated inside the labia majora. They are likewise shrouded in pubic hair.

Uterus: The uterus is a pear-formed organ that is situated between the bladder and the rectum. It is where a child is created during pregnancy.

Ovaries: The ovaries are the female contraceptive organs. They produce eggs and estrogen, the female sex chemical.

Fallopian tubes: The fallopian tubes are two cylinders that interface the ovaries to the uterus. They convey eggs from the ovaries to the uterus.

Sexual reaction in various societies

Sexual reaction is a general human encounter, however, the way that individuals experience and express sexual joy changes from one culture to another. In certain societies, sex is transparently examined and celebrated, while in different societies, being a confidential matter is thought of. There is no set-in-stone manner to encounter sexual joy, and it is essential to be deferential to the various ways that individuals express their sexuality.

Conclusion

Sexual reaction is an intricate and interesting interaction that is impacted by various variables, including science, brain research, and culture. Understanding sexual reactions can assist us with bettering grasping ourselves and our accomplices. It can likewise assist us with conveying all the more about our

sexual requirements and wants.

Chapter6:

Body, soul, and Love

The faculties and erotic nature are personally entwined with human life systems, assuming a significant part in our capacity to encounter and draw in with our general surroundings. Our five detects - sight, hearing, contact, taste, and smell - furnish us with a steady stream of tangible data that assists us with grasping our current circumstances, interfacing with others, and valuing the magnificence and intricacy of the world.

Sight: Sight is maybe the most predominant of our faculties, permitting us to see the world in energetic detail. The eyes, with their many-sided organization of photoreceptors and brain associations, catch the light and change it into electrical signs that are shipped off the cerebrum for understanding. Through sight, we can recognize varieties, shapes, and examples, and we can see profundity and development. Sight permits us to see the value in the magnificence of nature, the complexities of craftsmanship and engineering, and the outflows of human inclination.

Hearing : Hearing is another fundamental sense that associates us with our general surroundings. Sound waves, going from the unobtrusive vibrations of a murmur to the strong thunder of thunder, are caught by our ears and changed over into electrical signs that are shipped off the cerebrum for understanding. Through hearing, we can recognize various pitches, volumes, and tones, and we can perceive the hints of discourse, music, and the climate. Hearing permits us to speak with others, partake in the tunes and harmonies of music, and value the hints of nature, from the trilling of birds to the crashing of waves.

Touch: Contact is the most personal of our faculties, permitting us to encounter the actual world in direct contact. The skin, with its huge organization of sensitive spots, is our essential organ of touch, fit for identifying pressure, temperature, surface, and torment. Through touch, we can investigate our general surroundings, and experience the glow of the sun on our skin, the non-abrasiveness of a bloom petal, or the harshness of bark. Contact permits us to communicate friendship, solace, and backing through motions like embraces and handshakes.

Taste: Taste is a perplexing sense that permits us to perceive the kind of food and drinks. The tongue, with its great many taste buds, is our essential organ of taste, fit for identifying sweet, harsh, pungent, unpleasant, and umami flavors. Taste assists us with recognizing nutritious food varieties, keeping away from harmful substances, and experiencing the huge swath of culinary enjoyments that various societies bring to the table.

Smell: Smell is a strong sense that can bring major areas of strength for out and recollections. The olfactory receptors, situated in the nasal cavity, distinguish smell particles in the air and convey messages to the cerebrum for translation. Through smell, we can recognize innumerable scents, from the lovely fragrance of newly heated bread to the sharp scent of newly cut grass. The smell can set off recollections of previous encounters, summon feelings like happiness or loathing, and even impact our way of behaving.

Sexiness and the Apprehensive System

The faculties assume an urgent part in our capacity to encounter exotic nature, which includes the elevated view of tangible upgrades and the related sensations of delight and satisfaction. At the point when we draw in with the world through our faculties, we enact brain processes in the mind that trigger the arrival of synapses like dopamine and endorphins. These synapses are related to sensations of joy, award, and prosperity.

The Job of Exotic Nature in Human Experience

Exotic nature is a fundamental part of human experience, permitting us to interface with our bodies, with others, and with our general surroundings. It improves our lives by upgrading our pleasure in food, music, workmanship, and nature. It cultivates closeness and association in our connections. Furthermore, it gives a wellspring of joy and self-disclosure.

Conclusion

The faculties and exotic nature are profoundly incorporated into human life systems, furnishing us with a rich and different tangible scene that shapes how we might interpret the world and our place inside it. Through our faculties, we experience the magnificence, intricacy, and marvel of life. What's more, through exotic nature, we track down delight, association, and satisfaction.

Impacts of love on an individual's well-being

Love has significant and broad consequences for an individual's prosperity. It can decidedly affect our actual well-being, emotional wellness, profound prosperity, and social connections.

Actual Health: Love has been displayed to emphatically affect our actual well-being. Studies have shown that individuals in cherishing connections will generally have lower levels of pressure chemicals, like cortisol, and more significant levels of resistant framework cells. Love can likewise assist with bringing down pulse, further develop rest quality, and lift energy levels.

Mental Health: Love is likewise gainful for our emotional wellness. Studies have shown that individuals with cherished connections will generally have lower levels of uneasiness and melancholy and more significant levels of confidence and joy. Love can likewise assist with decreasing pressure, working on mental capability, and lifting flexibility notwithstanding affliction.

Close to home Well-being: Love is a central human need, and when we feel cherished and upheld, we feel more associated with others and to ourselves. This can prompt expanded close-to-home prosperity, which is described by sensations of bliss, fulfilment, and reason. Love can likewise assist with buffering us from gloomy feelings, like pity, outrage, and dejection.

Social Relationships: Love is fundamental for building and keeping up with solid social connections. At the point when we feel cherished and upheld by others, we are bound to trust, coordinate, and be empathetic towards others. This can prompt more grounded social associations, which are related with a great many advantages, including joy, life span, and lower levels of pressure and melancholy.

Conclusion

Love is a strong power that can significantly affect our prosperity. It can work on our actual wellbeing, emotional wellness, profound prosperity, and social connections. In a world that can frequently feel cold and separated, love gives us a feeling of having a place, security, and reason. It is a gift that we ought to value and sustain, as it is perhaps of the main purpose to calculate our general well-being and bliss.

Chapter7:

Anatomy Behind Yearning

The Organic Underpinnings of Sexuality and Longing

Our organic cosmetics play a significant part in molding our sexual encounters. Chemicals, like testosterone, estrogen, and oxytocin, impact our sexual drive, excitement, and holding. These chemicals are delivered by different organs in the body and follow up on various pieces of the mind, incorporating regions engaged with remuneration, inspiration, and feeling.

The sensory system likewise assumes a basic part in sexuality. An intricate organisation of nerves and synapses is liable for communicating signals between the mind, privates, and different pieces of the body. These signs are fundamental for sexual excitement, climax, and sexual delight.

Mental Variables Affecting Sexuality and Longing: Mental variables, including our contemplations, feelings, and encounters, likewise significantly affect our sexuality. Our confidence, self-perception, and past sexual encounters can all impact our sexual cravings and ways of behaving.

Longing: specifically, is a complex mental peculiarity that is well-established in our feelings and encounters. It is frequently connected with sensations of want, yearning, and deficiency. Longing can be coordinated towards someone else, a particular sexual demonstration, or a more summed-up feeling of closeness or satisfaction.

The Transaction of Science and Brain Research in Human Sexuality

The organic and mental elements that impact human sexuality are not independent substances; they are unpredictably entwined. Our chemicals and synapses can impact our contemplations, feelings, and ways of behaving, and our mental encounters can, thus, influence our chemical levels and mind actions.

This exchange between science and brain research is clear in the experience of longing. Longing can be set off by natural elements, like hormonal changes or actual boosts, yet it is additionally molded by our mental state, including our assumptions, wants, and profound connections.

Self-excitement and Sexual Longing: A Complex Relationship

Self-excitement: the demonstration of invigorating oneself physically, is a typical and regular human way of behaving. It very well may be a wellspring of joy, unwinding, and self-revelation. Be that as it may, self-excitement can likewise be a wellspring of disarray, uneasiness, and responsibility, especially when it is joined by extraordinary sexual longing.

Sexual longing: a profound yearning for sexual closeness and satisfaction, is a strong close-to-home expression that can rouse us to search out sexual encounters. While sexual longing can be coordinated towards an accomplice, it can likewise appear as a craving for self-excitement.

The connection between self-excitement and sexual longing is intricate and complex. From one perspective, self-excitement can assist with lightening sexual pressure and longing, giving a feeling of delivery and satisfaction. Then again, self-excitement can likewise increase sexual longing, making a pattern of want and disappointment.

The Mental Impacts of Self-arousal

Self-excitement can significantly affect our considerations, feelings, and ways of behaving. It can build our sexual craving, excitement, and dream action. It can likewise prompt changes in temperament, like expanded sensations of energy, joy, and unwinding.

At times, self-excitement can likewise set off gloomy feelings, like culpability, nervousness, and disgrace. This is especially liable to happen assuming an individual accepts that self-excitement is off-base or undesirable.

The Impacts of Self-excitement on Sexual Yearning

Self-excitement can affect sexual longing. On the positive side, it can assist with lessening sexual pressure and give a feeling of satisfaction. This can, thus, make it simpler to oversee sexual longing and spotlight on different parts of life.

On the negative side, self-excitement can likewise strengthen sexual longing, creating a pattern of want and dissatisfaction. This is on the grounds that self-excitement can build the degree of excitement in the body, which can make it harder to zero in on different exercises or connections.

Solid Self-excitement Practices:

Self-excitement can be a sound and charming piece of an individual's sexual life. In any case, moving toward it in a careful and mindful way is significant. Here are a few hints for solid self-excitement rehearses:

Know about your motivations: Wonder why you are participating in self-excitement. Could it be said that you are involving it as a method for easing sexual strain, investigating your sexuality, or interfacing with your body? Having a reasonable comprehension of your inspirations can assist you with making solid decisions.

Set boundaries. Conclude how long and energy you need to spend on self-excitement. It is likewise essential to define limits around what you are OK with and what you are not.

Practice mindfulness: Focus on your viewpoints, feelings, and sensations during self-excitement. This can assist you with better grasping your body and your sexual reactions.

Utilise self-excitement as a device for self-discovery. Explore different avenues regarding various strategies and investigate what feels better to you. This can assist you with fostering your very own superior comprehension of sexuality.

Looking for Proficient Help?:

Assuming you are battling with self-excitement or sexual longing, looking for proficient help is significant. A specialist can assist you with figuring out the foundation of your interests and foster sound survival strategies

Adverse consequences

Responsibility and disgrace: A few people might encounter culpability or disgrace related to self-excitement. This can be because of social or strict convictions, or individual qualities that view self-excitement as negative.

Addiction: At times, self-excitement can become exorbitant or enthusiastic, prompting habit. This can slow down day-to-day existence, connections, and work or studies.

Overstimulation: Unreasonable self-excitement can prompt overstimulation and desensitization, making it hard to encounter sexual delight with an accomplice.

Distraction: Self-excitement can turn into an interruption from other significant parts of life, like connections, work, or side interests.

Actual inconvenience: Now and again, self-excitement can prompt actual inconvenience, like torment or aggravation.

By and large, the impacts of self-excitement are mind-boggling and differ from one individual to another. A few people might encounter for the most part constructive outcomes, while others might encounter generally pessimistic impacts. It is essential to be aware of one's own encounters and to look for proficient assistance if self-excitement is creating issues in one's day-to-day existence.

Conclusion

Self-excitement and sexual longing are complicated and complex peculiarities. They can be a wellspring of joy, fervor, and self-revelation. Notwithstanding, they can likewise be a wellspring of disarray, uneasiness, and culpability. Moving toward self-excitement in a careful and mindful way is significant. In the event that you are battling with self-excitement or sexual longing, kindly look for proficient assistance.

www.ingramcontent.com/pod-product-compliance
Lightning Source LLC
Chambersburg PA
CBHW070951260726
48661CB00003B/1229